First Edition published January, 2016

ISBN-13: 978-1523303632

ISBN-10: 1523303638

To those who live with chronic pain or are loving
someone who does

~~~~~~

Special thanks to the ones who already understood me
before I wrote this book

"You don't look like there's anything wrong with you!" I could write an entire novella on that misunderstanding alone. But I choose to develop it here in the introduction rather than dwell on this particularly ignorant supposition. I do not use the word ignorant as a slam. How could someone who feels well possibly understand that all is not always well that looks well? They have no experience with such a state. And this particular group is one of my target audiences. This is written to teach, illuminate and explain, not retaliate or reprove. I have chosen to discuss five misunderstandings although I feel certain there are many more.

As odd as it might seem, and perhaps I'm not the only one to have had the thought, I have often longed for a cane or a wheelchair. Never for the sake of drawing attention to oneself, but something to alert others that I am not functioning at the level they are or that I wish I could or, better yet, that I appear to be. Something to instantly trigger their understanding of a health problem is needed here. But if I had that visible aid then I wouldn't be a true Silent Paper Doll. I would have no knowledge to share on such a tricky topic of a seemingly invisible health issue.

I have chosen the image of a paper doll for several reasons. Those of you who played with them as a child remember the fragility of their materials. They were easily torn if great care was not taken. Also, the child was the decision maker of what the doll would wear. They dressed the doll as they thought best in an array of choices. There were literally dozens, if not hundreds, of clothing designs anything from fancy dress coats and sunglasses to swimwear and business suits. In the end, the child had determined the visual state of its doll. And nothing looks sharper than a lovely paper doll. There is almost always a smile on the doll's face and if it had any emotions they are buried deep in paper stock. Paper dolls are lifeless and can exist in only one dimension. I think it's fair to say those with chronic pain feel they are living only part of a life, particularly in comparison to others. And this gives the lives of others the illusion of fanciful fairy tales.

The adult world tends to behave towards someone suffering with chronic pain as the child I described above. They look at the outside and perceive with their eyes that no problem exists. After all, that cane and wheelchair are nowhere to be found. And the one with chronic pain is doing their best to silently hold it all together. So no wonder the misunderstandings exist.

As much as I would like, I cannot remove pain from people's lives. I cannot tell you what are the best options for the chronic pain situation you or your loved one faces. This I have to leave to the professionals. I can, however, relate my personal experiences and heartfelt thoughts. My hope is someone might be helped and encouraged, whatever their role in these debilitating circumstances.

I referred to my Paper Dolls as being silent because for the most part they don't speak about their pain, except to fellow sojourners. They don't want to dwell on or explain their pain to others. Experience has taught and shown trying to explain is not fruitful. And the more it's talked about and discussed the more real and…painful it all becomes. So they won't always tell you when they're hurting but chances will be that they always are.

I considered sharing how I came to be on my particular path of pain. It will soon be 19 of my 44 years. But I do not want the attention to be on my exact story. I doubt that others want the focus to be on their exact stories either. What someone in pain is undoubtedly seeking from you is nothing more than simply your compassionate understanding. And that I believe is the most powerful gift you can give them.

For when I am weak, He is very strong.

The Apostle Paul

NUMBER ONE
~ ATTENTION DOLL ~

It's vital to establish that I have many people in my life who also suffer with chronic pain. After almost two decades one naturally finds themselves meeting others in the same circumstances. This again makes me no expert, but I certainly can speak from a broad base of experience.

As for myself and of those I know, I can fervently state that not one has imagined, pretended or wished themselves into a life with chronic pain. Perhaps those types of situations do exist but not on my plane. And yes sadly I have heard through the years many a time that people with chronic pain are seeking attention. Never confuse seeking understanding with seeking attention! All of that being said, the very sad irony is pain does require much attention. And from the person in pain's perspective it is negative attention.

I think of all the ways one could receive positive attention. Let your mind sit there for a moment....a successful career, family activities, memorable time spent with friends, use of talents...the list is very long. Someone living with true chronic pain did not choose to forego those means of joy. Never in a million years.

Of all the misunderstandings this one is no doubt the most painful to process. If you are hoping to show compassion for someone in pain, believing they are only seeking the world's attention is not the way to do it!

NUMBER TWO
~ LAZY DOLL ~

Here we find another classic. I can think of nothing sillier than choosing a life of having to lie down or get extra rest due to severe pain. Who wouldn't rather be active and constructive with their time? Who would spend money ad infinitum on physical therapy and other treatments if the need was not there? I would rather have a pair of fun shoes now and then myself.

People with chronic pain are often unable to work and that is rarely by choice. So be very careful with this one. Guilt abounds in a home where money is in short supply and someone with pain is unable to work. Not to mention that loss of positive contribution one can experience which I mentioned earlier. I believe that God placed a desire in all of us to produce and be a part of this life. Depending on the degree of a pain on any given day, those goals are near impossible.

Time and energies transition from a busy work week schedule to a busy doctor/therapy schedule. Chronic pain sufferers may have as many as five practitioner visits every week simply as a maintenance program. Never allow yourself to think of them as bonbon eaters watching re-runs of Oprah. A pain plan schedule is challenging to coordinate.

Oh and if only I had a dollar for every time I was told to exercise and do more strength training. Sadly strength training is something most in pain would love to be able to do. But exercise/strength training can often aggravate pain symptoms and then a vicious circle begins to swirl. "No pain no gain" may work for some, but not for all.

NUMBER THREE
~ ISOLATION DOLL ~

Most with chronic pain can remember a time in their lives when things were quite different. They were active and able to do so much more. Now they find themselves basing many, if not all, decisions on how a circumstance is going to affect their pain. It could range from the comfort of a restaurant chair, church pew, or to a hotel room bed.

After years pass, the walls of pain close in to form a cage and pain becomes just that, a cage. Gone are the trips, dinners out and hosting parties. Quiet private time now has to take their place. It is never a happy thing to turn down friends or family who would like to go out and have "normal" recreational events. In fact a chronic pain sufferer misses the interaction they once had but, at the same time, knows they must balance and weigh everything based on how it is going to affect their pain level. It is often the case that pain becomes an insurmountable fear.

Never doubt you are still valued and play an important role in their life. But the role is changed, just as it has for the one living in pain.

NUMBER FOUR
~ CRAZY DOLL ~

Keeping a healthy mind balance with chronic pain is a challenge and one I can only even begin to accomplish with my faith, a team of physical therapists, chiropractors, massage, etc. and the irrevocable support of those who love me. But years of pressure on your body does take a toll on your mind. People can misinterpret this as being an airhead. Tears are a normal part of chronic pain and those can be misinterpreted as being off balance or "crazy." Remember that someone with pain is literally struggling to get through a day. Basic daily functions become challenging depending on level of pain. I find myself not remembering things that I know I know. Obviously, someone in pain is still intelligent and has valid thoughts. But pain can cloud thinking. There is a multitude of helpful information from the medical field regarding the effects on the brain from chronic pain. There is also a multitude of discouraging information from the medical field. Ranging from "it's all in your head" to "you'll just have to learn to live with the pain," doctors do their best to diagnose one of the more illusive health problems. Imagine being told "it's all in your head" when the pain is so real you can never escape it. Better yet, imagine arriving at the emergency room with classic stroke or heart attack symptoms and being told "it's all in your head." It's very disconcerting to say the least.

Sure, your loved one may have changed from who they once were, but they are far from crazy. Please be sure you are not adding to that stigma.

NUMBER FIVE
~ FLAKY DOLL ~

Normal. Now that is a word that is both a burden and a blessing. A burden because it cannot be achieved and a blessing because one still longs to. Sadly I have lost friendships and relationships simply because I never know how my body is going to feel at any given time. Therefore, reliability becomes a huge problem.

Someone might invite me to lunch and I agree and then the time comes and it's what we with pain call a "bad day." Bad days are the ones when plans get changed because the pain is too great. They can range from staying in bed all day in a dark room to not being well enough to get ready to go out into the world. Someone who understands this is priceless to those living in a pain cage!

Pain requires maximum amounts of flexibility because you are always in flux. "Good days" are rare and far between. Those are the days groceries can be gotten and even then it is a difficult task albeit mundane for others. Typing at the computer, reading, sitting, all of these things are taken for granted but not by someone in pain. Those can be luxuries on a "good day" or impossibilities on a "bad day."

THE TRUTH
~ BURDEN DOLL ~

After discussing the misunderstood dolls it only seems right to develop the doll of reality. It's not easy to describe how much guilt a person in pain allows to weigh on them. We fall very short in so many areas, unable to meet people's expectations and hopes. The disappointment on loved one's faces is hard to carry if a visit for pain treatment didn't go well. (Sometimes they just don't for whatever reasons, another variable that exists.) We want so very badly to be well, sometimes more for others than even ourselves. Although we may not be considered burdens to be cared for, we certainly feel that we are. I think most of us would much prefer to be able to care for others, meet their needs rather than them having to do that for us. I have aging parents and live with the constant anxiety of how I will care for them to the degree they have cared for me. There is so much in my heart to give that my body doesn't allow. I know I speak for many in that last statement.

On a happy note, people in pain have been freed from the illusion of "independence." They had to learn to rely on others at some point, both a necessity and a nuisance. It may have happened gradually or quite suddenly. The simplest of tasks became frustrations that are nigh impossible to complete. People are at so many different levels. Sadly, many will stay in their state all the remaining days this side of Eternity. They will never push a grocery cart without feeling pain or read a book curled up on the couch again. Gone is recreation where the atmosphere can't be carefully predicted. Everything becomes this controlled zone to limit pain to any degree possible. In some ridiculous turn about, that pain cage actually evolved into a safe place.

And, for some, there are no others to assist them with the demands of every day life. Wouldn't that be the most terrible situation of all, to journey this road alone? I am thinking of a specific friend as I type those words. She is a single mom raising a precious autistic son. The mental image that always comes to mind is a juggler trying to juggle life with not one hand, but no hands. She is a hero.

And I suppose we are all heroes in some bizarre way. Thank you for reading these thoughts. I leave you with this final one. May we not cause the ones with chronic pain to experience more pain!

Those of you who have either the fortune, or misfortune, of knowing me personally know that I love a good fairy tale. And I love a happy ending. In fact, this is usually the content of most of my writings. There aren't a lot of happy endings for people with pain.

But, that being said…

ONCE UPON A TIME there lived a young woman who was ambitious and proud. She had goals set and plans made to establish her place in the kingdom. And in that kingdom lived a young man who too was a bit ambitious and proud. He had goals set and plans made to lead a simple life doing work he loved.

Their paths would collide on a fateful day. Neither more mystified by the resplendence of the other. They had met their match and were soon married. Some people in the kingdom did not approve and misjudged their magical beginning. But the couple was indeed one in soul and spirit, their hearts intertwined in such a unique way. Years passed and joy and fun abounded. But soon the road narrowed and pain entered into the castle of love they shared. Doctors were sought and brought by the dozens but her pain could not be eradicated. Everything had forever changed yet their love burned strong.

One day the young man, who is not as young as he once was, brought to his bride what would become a symbol of joy. It was called The Princess Ring. It would represent all the many things of beauty that the couple would not experience in the future. Others in the kingdom still traveled, dined and raised families, those sorts of things. But this would not be for them. God had another path for them to walk together. Still to this day the young woman, who is not as young as she once was, wears this ring and remembers the pledge of love she received when her husband placed it on her finger. There is no pain too great to separate her from her husband's love or God's love for her!

THE END